Organic Lip Balms Quick Start Guide

Rejuvenate & Protect your Lips with Natural Homemade Lip Balm Recipes

Table of Contents

Introduction

I want to thank you and congratulate you for purchasing the book, *"Organic Lip Balms Quick Start Guide: Rejuvenate & Protect Your Lips with Natural Homemade Lip Balm Recipes".*

This book contains proven steps and strategies on how to make your own homemade lip balms using safe and organic ingredients.

Lip balms are important for the care and protection of the lips. While it is possible to buy organic lip balms in the stores nowadays, there is an advantage in making your own. First, you can personalize it according to your needs, desired flavor and even tint. Second, since you are in control of your recipes, you can be sure that your product is completely organic and does not contain any ingredients you are allergic or sensitive to. Third, it is so much fun to make your own. You can even give away your homemade lip balms as gifts or sell them.

Thanks again for purchasing this book, I hope you enjoy it!

Chapter 1 – The Basics – What is a Lip Balm?

Before anything else, you must know the basics of making your own personal products. Some of you may already have experience in making your own skin care products, but for those who are complete beginners, the first two chapters are must-reads.

First, what is a lip balm? A lip balm is an emollient substance which is used to moisturize, protect and/or rejuvenate the lips. Depending on the ingredients used in your lip balm, one product can do all three or you can make three separate products for each purpose.

The terms 'moisturize,' 'protect' and 'rejuvenate' are sometimes used vaguely by lip balm manufacturers because they may argue that whatever is moisturizing is also protecting and rejuvenating, and vice versa. However, since you would likely want to personalize your lip balms, you need to know a clear definition of these terms.

To moisturize means to add moisture to parched or dry lips. The lips are considered part of the skin, but they are thinner than other skin areas and don't contain oil and sweat glands. In other areas of the skin, sebum or the skin's natural oil provides some degree of protection from the natural elements. Sebum provides a sun protection factor (SPF) of 6 to 8, and it prevents dryness.

Of course, it does not provide enough protection from the harsh sun and extreme temperatures, but the point is it still provides some protection for the skin. The lips, on the other hand, have no natural protection at all, which is why they are usually dry even in people with naturally oily skin.

Moisturizing ingredients for lip balms are similar to those used in skin moisturizers except for one crucial requirement: they must not be poisonous when consumed in tiny amounts. Since lip balms are applied on the lips, the ingredients can inevitably be consumed in the process of eating, talking, pressing the lips together and licking the lips.

While lip balms are not foods and should not be consumed in large amounts (for doing so might be dangerous), the ingredients should pose no danger when only a very small amount is consumed. The same requirement applies to other ingredients that protect and rejuvenate.

In chapter 3, we will discuss the various moisturizing ingredients you can use for your lip balms.

Protecting ingredients are those that protect the lips from the natural elements like the sun, extreme temperatures, wind, pollution, and so on. The difference between moisturizing ingredients and protecting ingredients is their primary purpose. The primary purpose of the former is to moisturize or to cure dry lips, while that of the latter is to protect the lips from the elements that may cause dryness.

On the surface, it may seem like these two are the same, but to make the point clear, here is an example: To moisturize the lips, plant-based oils like coconut oil or olive oil may be used. These ingredients are readily absorbed by dry lips; however, once they are absorbed, they provide no protection from the sun or wind. You can opt to apply more when your lips get dry again, but to avoid that nuisance, you can add protective ingredients that lock out the elements causing dryness. An example of such an ingredient is beeswax.

You might think that beeswax is also a moisturizing ingredient, and you are correct in thinking this. However, since it is a wax, it will be absorbed slower in comparison to oils. If your lips are very dry and you need a quick relief, wax is not the best solution. Further, if your lips are chapped and look ugly, applying wax will exacerbate the problem because it will get around the edges of the chapped parts and make them look more obvious.

Depending on your specific lip problem, you may need to use a separate product to moisturize and another one to protect. If you are not going outdoors, a moisturizing product may be enough. If your lips are not overly dry but you are heeded outdoors, a protecting product may be enough. If your lips are very dry and chapped and you need to be outdoors, you may need two separate products. If you are very active and don't have time to reapply, you may need one product with both ingredients. The possibilities are endless. They will be discussed further in the succeeding chapters.

In chapter 4, we will discuss the various protecting ingredients you can use depending on the effect you wish to achieve.

Lastly, rejuvenating ingredients are those that stimulate or help the lips' skin cells to repair themselves; thus, allowing the lips to remain younger-looking for longer. Again, it is possible to say that moisturizing and protecting ingredients can also be considered rejuvenating ingredients because the former keeps the lips looking younger and the latter prevents the elements from damaging the lips. However, following the explanation given above, rejuvenating ingredients are those whose primary purpose is to repair the lips. These ingredients are similar to those used in organic anti-aging skin care.

In chapter 5 we will discuss the various rejuvenating ingredients you can use for anti-aging lip care.

Chapter 2 – The Basics – DIY Tools and Rules

If you wish to make your own skin care products like do-it-yourself lip balms, then you must have specific tools to make your work easier. You must also follow some basic rules to ensure safety and cleanliness.

First, regarding the tools, you don't need to kit yourself with a professional chemist's tools, but you do need some specific items. Since lip balms may contain waxes that need to be melted, you must have some tools for this. A microwaveable bowl or small sauce pan will do. Since lip balms, though edible in small amounts, are not food, it is best to set aside this bowl or saucepan specifically for the making of lip balms.

You also need a tool for mixing the lip balm ingredients. A metal spoon set aside for this purpose is sufficient, but you can also use disposable wooden popsicle sticks or wooden chopsticks. Do not reuse these sticks since the ingredients will soak into them and may contaminate your other batches of lip balms.

As much as possible, do not use your fingers for mixing. The hot melted wax may burn you and you may contaminate the lip balm with germs. If you insist on using your fingers, then make sure your hands are clean including under the fingernails. Contaminated organic lip balms will spoil easily since they do not contain commercial preservatives.

The containers for your finished product must also be included in your tool kit. If you don't need a lip balm for outdoors, you can just keep your product in any covered container, but it will obviously be inconvenient for travel. The most convenient and familiar lip balm container is the plastic lip balm tube. You can purchase it wholesale from specialty stores. You need to wash them in soapy water first to remove any impurities then dry them completely.

If you choose to use these, you might need a dropper or pipette to fill them up or else make sure that your hands are very steady. Droppers or pipettes for making DIY skin care can also be purchased from specialty shops. Afterwards, the filled tubes can be covered with labels if you wish to give away your lip balms or sell them.

It is not advisable to reuse lip balm tubes because they are not that durable. The twist screw may no longer work due to constant use and it can be difficult to completely clean them of old lip balm residue. At any rate, since they are cheap, it will not be difficult to rebuy them. If you are worried about the waste, buy from sellers who use recycled plastic and recycle your used tubes as well.

The second most familiar lip balm container is the metal or plastic pot. These come in all shapes and sizes, but fastidious people dislike them because they need to use their finger to apply the lip balm and the residue must be wiped off from the finger afterwards. Of course, the decision regarding which container to use is up to you. Lip balm pots must also be washed and dried before use. If they are not damaged, you can recycle them because they can be easily cleaned of old lip balm residues.

Second, regarding the rules on handling ingredients, they must be treated like food to avoid spoilage and contamination. It is best to buy only small amounts of ingredients at a time and to keep them in a cool dark place. If you live in a hot climate, it might be better to keep your ingredients in the refrigerator. Discard anything that doesn't smell or look as it should.

Chapter 3 – The Ingredients – Moisture

As discussed in the first chapter, these ingredients have the primary purpose of providing moisture to dry lips. While they can also protect or rejuvenate the lips, they work best as moisturizers.

The quickest acting lip moisturizers are plant oils like coconut, olive, sunflower, and the like. In fact, if your lips are perpetually parched and you need instant relief, the best solution is to dab a small amount of any of these oils directly onto the lips then wait a few seconds to facilitate full absorption. You can keep these oils in a small, spill-proof container.

The kind of oil you choose will depend on how dry your lips are and your personal preference since plant oils have their own scent and taste. Coconut and olive oils are generally best for very dry lips. Argan oil is also a good choice but it can be more expensive. If you prefer a neutral smelling and tasting oil, try grape seed, peanut or canola oil.

If this discussion is starting to sound like this book is about food, don't worry. Most of the ingredients used in organic skin care are also used in cooking; thus, there is no need to buy a separate bottle of olive oil for making lip balms if you already have a bottle for cooking use. Some books will advise that you must use cosmetic grade oils for making organic skin care, but there is really no need for that.

Legally speaking, food grade cooking oils are safer because they are meant to be ingested. Cosmetic grade oils are only tested safe for topical application. Since lip balms are used on the lips and can be easily ingested in small amounts, it is better to stick with food grade ingredients. Besides, they are generally cheaper in comparison to cosmetic grade ingredients because they do not come in fancy packaging.

If you already have cosmetic grade oils like castor or jojoba oils, then you can use these too. These oils are inedible so they are only used for skin care and other topical purposes. The point here is you don't have to go out and buy new supplies just to make lip balm. You can use whatever you already have. However, if you wish to stick to using natural and safe ingredients for your organic lip balms, avoid using mineral oil and petroleum jelly since these are not natural. They are the residues after refining crude oil.

Another moisturizing ingredient for lip balms is emollient wax like Shea butter and cocoa butter. These waxes are soft and melt easily, making them readily absorbed by the lips. Since they are waxes, they leave a thin film of wax on the lips; thus, providing some protection, but they are more moisturizing than protecting.

You can use these moisturizing ingredients alone or mix them with other lip balm ingredients. Using these ingredients alone will provide maximum moisture to the lips, but they can be inconvenient while traveling. Plant oils are liquid and can spill, and emollient waxes, though solid can melt easily. Also, since they provide no or very little protection from natural elements that dry the lips, they need to be constantly reapplied.

To make a more solid and more protective product, these ingredients are usually mixed with harder waxes like beeswax, but the more moisturizing lip balms will most likely be on the soft side due to the higher percentage of moisturizing ingredients.

You can check out sample recipes for moisturizing lip balms in chapter 7.

Chapter 4 – The Ingredients - Protection

The primary purpose of ingredients that protect the lips is to provide a shield from the natural elements that may dry out the thin and fragile lip skin. Thus, these ingredients must be those that are not readily absorbed. Generally speaking, the harder the wax is or the less easily it melts, the more protective it can be for the lips.

Beeswax was already mentioned as an example of such an ingredient. This provides a great honey smell and taste to your lip balm. Another example is candelilla wax. This wax is cheap, making it a common ingredient in most inexpensive commercial lip balms. However, too much of it can make the lip balm too waxy, i.e. it leaves a thick layer of wax on the lips which can feel uncomfortable and look ugly particularly on very dry and chapped lips. While waxy lip balms provide long-lasting protection from the elements, they are not that moisturizing.

Pure hard waxes alone cannot be used as a lip balm because they are solid and cannot be spread. You must melt them first and mix with a moisturizing ingredient. To make a protective lip balm, more hard wax is used than oil or emollient wax. It is best to start with a ratio of 3 parts hard wax with 2 parts oil or emollient wax.

Depending on the quality of hard wax you have, you may need to add less. The resulting lip balm should be solid once cooled but still soft enough to spread on the lips. Once on the lips, the waxy layer should be thick enough to provide protection but thin enough to not be too obvious and look ugly. The lips should feel like they are coated with product, but their natural color should still be visible.

For those who are often exposed to the sun, hard waxes provide an SFP of 15. This should be enough for normal use, but for those who require higher SPF, carrot seed oil provides an SPF of at least 38 and raspberry seed oil provides at least 28. At least 1 tablespoon of oil must be used per 1 teaspoon of hard wax. Using these seed oils gives the advantage of making the lip balm less waxy and more moisturizing; however, in being more emollient they are more easily absorbed and must be reapplied often compared to the more waxy balms.

You can check out sample recipes for protective lip balms in chapter 7.

Chapter 5 – The Ingredients – Rejuvenation

The ingredients for rejuvenation are primarily used to stimulate and help the lips' skin cells to repair themselves. The lips are among the first parts of the face to show age especially if they are constantly exposed to the sun. While SPF will lessen the sun's aging effects, the natural process of aging will still have an effect on the look of your lips. When this happens, they will benefit from additional rejuvenating ingredients.

The most common rejuvenating ingredients used in all natural lip balms are essential oils and plant oils. Peppermint or cinnamon essential oils stimulate blood flow to the lips; thus, bringing in more nutrients and oxygen to the skin cells. Having more nutrients and oxygen means these cells have an easier time repairing themselves.

In addition, peppermint or cinnamon oil taste great, freshen the breath and slightly plump the lips thus giving them an attractive look. Lavender essential oil also works the same way, but some people may dislike the taste. However, those who like lavender flavored desserts will find lavender lip balm unique and sophisticated.

If you dislike the plumping effect of peppermint, cinnamon or lavender (perhaps because your lips are already plump or too sensitive), you can try rose essential oil which provides nutrients and antioxidants necessary for skin repair. If the taste and smell of rose are too cloying, try mixing it with some other flavor. If you prefer fruity tastes, orange or grapefruit essential oils are worth trying. If your lips are dark due to the sun or too much smoking, lemon essential oil will gradually lighten them.

You can also mix the essential oils to get several benefits in one lip balm. Just take note of the resulting flavor and scent. Some tried and tested but still unique flavor combinations include rose and lemon, and peppermint and grapefruit.

To provide a rejuvenating effect and not just a hint of flavor, add at least 1 drop of essential oil per 1 gram of lip balm. A regular lip balm tube will contain at least 4 grams of lip balm, so it is best to use a total of 4 drops of essential oil, but take note that this is the *total* amount of essential oil. If you use combinations like rose and lemon, two drops of each will give a balanced flavor, but of course, if you prefer it to be more lemony, you can use 3 drops of lemon and 1 drop of rose.

On the subject of essential oils, it is important to use only those that are safe for ingestion. Some essential oils are poisonous, e.g. tea tree oil and neem oil, and must never be used in any kind of lip product. Also, since you will inevitably taste and smell these oils, use only those that you can tolerate. For example, frankincense is a good essential oil for anti-aging, and you can safely use it for lip balms. However, if using it makes you feel like you are eating your grandmother's perfume, you will likely end up not using it and thus wasting your product.

Further, make sure to use only true essential oils and not artificial fragrance oils. The latter are oils to which artificial fragrance has been added. They can be irritating even to non-sensitive skins and are dangerous when ingested. If you are not sure what you are buying, always check the label and only buy from reputable sources. The label should state the scientific name of the plant, its country of origin and date of manufacture. It should also indicate that the contents are 100% essential oil.

If the label does not provide all these information, do not buy that brand. For more information on essential oils and how to use them safely, please check out other books or websites. Alternatively, you can just stick with the suggestions given above.

If you would rather not use essential oils, you can use plant oils with anti-aging properties like argan oil and rosehip oil. These are particularly high in antioxidants and nutrients that are good for skin repair. Since these ingredients are also very emollient, you can consider them as both moisturizing and rejuvenating ingredients. The other moisturizing plant oils like olive and coconut can also provide some anti-aging benefits due to their antioxidant content, but their benefits lean more towards their moisturizing effect. Argan and rosehip oils are more expensive, but when used pure on the lips or as the sole moisturizing oil in a lip balm, they will provide the most benefits.

Rejuvenating ingredients are best added to lip balms meant to be used at night because this is the time when your lips are repairing themselves. Also, since the lips are not exposed to the elements at night, you can opt to leave out protective ingredients. This will allow you to use more moisturizing and rejuvenating ingredients which, after soaking into the lips for 8 hours, will give you super soft lips.

To maximize the absorption of rejuvenating ingredients, it is best to exfoliate your lips first. You can easily do this by lightly brushing the lips with a toothbrush, or using a lip scrub made from a mixture of oil and sugar.

You can try the sample recipes for rejuvenating lip balms and lip scrubs in chapter 7.

Chapter 6 – The Extras

It is possible to use lip balms for basic purposes like moisturizing, protecting or rejuvenating the lips, but with the addition of extra ingredients like tint and shimmer, you can also use them as lip cosmetics. Also, you can add more flavors to make them more fun to use.

First, regarding tint, organic options include beetroot powder for red or pink tinted lip balms, alkanet root powder for more purplish shades, and cocoa powder or cinnamon for nude or brownish shades. These ingredients will add a slight flavor to your lip balm. If you want to keep the flavor neutral, you can try using organic food colorings.

It takes trial and error to determine how much coloring ingredient you need to use to achieve your desired tint. Start with a small amount of tint and check the effect by applying the cooled balm on your lips. If you want to add more tint, reheat the mixture to melt it and add more color. Take note of the final amount so you will get the same tint the next time you make a new batch.

Second, regarding shimmer, use mica powder that is specifically marketed for cosmetic use. Some mica powders are also tinted. You can add a similar tint of mica as your tinting ingredient to make the color deeper, or use a complementary color to make your lip balm look more sophisticated. For example, adding copper mica to red tinted lip balm will give a pretty effect.

Third, regarding flavor, the ingredients mentioned in the previous chapters will already give your lip balm subtle flavor, e.g. beeswax has a slight honey flavor, but you can still add other ingredients to intensify the taste. Organic options include natural flavor extracts, essential oils, and honey or a bit of powdered sugar for sweetness. Do not use granulated sugar since it might not melt completely, thereby resulting to a rough lip balm. The most common flavors for lip balms are sweet ones, but if you are adventurous, try a savory flavor like bacon.

Start with the sample recipes for tinted, shimmer and flavored lip balms in Chapter 7 then experiment with your own combinations afterwards.

Chapter 7 – Recipe Book for All Natural Lip Balm

These are sample recipes you can start with if you are completely new to making your own lip balms. Once you get the hang of it, try experimenting to come up with unique combinations. Each recipe will yield about 24 grams of lip balm which is enough to fill 5 regular tubes. However, the liquid lip oils must be stored in spill-proof bottles while less solid lip glosses are best stored in spill-proof pots.

Also, these recipes use organic ingredients and do not use preservatives. As a result, the products may spoil more readily than commercial lip products. If you will not use the finished products immediately, store them in the refrigerator; or else make smaller batches that you can use within 2 to 3 months.

Basic recipes

Moisturizing lip balm

3 tablespoons oil of your choice (coconut, olive, sunflower, etc.)

2 teaspoons emollient wax (cocoa butter, shea butter, etc.)

Heat the wax and oil together over low heat or in the microwave using the lowest setting. When melted, stir together then pour into your desired containers.

Protective lip balm

2 tablespoons oil of your choice

3 teaspoons beeswax or candelilla wax pellets

Follow the same procedure described above.

Moisturizing lip balm with SPF

1 tablespoon oil of your choice

2 tablespoons carrot seed oil or raspberry seed oil

2 teaspoons beeswax or candelilla wax pellets

Heat the wax and oil first, then mix well. When the mixture is slightly cool, add the seed oil. Mix again then pour into your containers.

Night rejuvenating lip oil

2 tablespoons argan or rosehip oil

10 drops of anti-aging essential oil (peppermint, cinnamon, lavender, lemon, orange, etc.)

Mix everything together in a spill proof bottle. Shake the bottle before use. Apply a small amount on the lips. Wait for the oil to be fully absorbed before sleeping.

Night rejuvenating lip balm

3 tablespoons argan or rosehip oil

2 teaspoons emollient wax

24 to 26 drops of anti-aging essential oil

Melt the wax and oil together. Let cool slightly then mix in the essential oil. Pour into your containers.

Moisturizing antioxidant lip balm

1 tablespoon coconut oil

1 tablespoon vitamin E oil

1 teaspoon beeswax pellets

Melt the beeswax and coconut oil together and mix well. Let cool slightly then add the vitamin E oil. Pour into your containers.

Lip plumping gloss

1 tablespoon neutral oil (grape seed, canola, jojoba, or castor)

½ teaspoon beeswax or candelilla wax pellets

5 drops peppermint or cinnamon essential oil

Melt the wax together with the oil and let cool slightly. Add the peppermint oil then pour into your containers, preferably a pot since this gloss is less solid than most lip balms. You can also add tint to this. (See below for tint ideas.)

Lip oil scrub

1 teaspoon oil of your choice

½ teaspoon granulated white or brown sugar

1 to 2 drops essential oil or natural flavor (optional)

Mix everything together in a bowl. Apply to the lips using light circular motions. Do not scrub lips for more than 1 minute. Rinse off. Apply rejuvenating lip oil or balm immediately.

Tinted lip balm or gloss

Make a batch of the basic moisturizing, basic protective or moisturizing with SPF lip balm recipe, then while the mixture is still hot, add the following ingredients depending on your desired tint. Mix well to ensure that the coloring ingredient is evenly distributed. Take note that these will only give a sheer tint, but you can always add more color if desired.

Pink: ½ teaspoon beetroot powder or 5 drops of natural liquid red food color

Red: ¾ to 1 teaspoon beetroot powder or 8 drops of natural liquid red food color

Maroon: ¼ teaspoon cinnamon and ½ teaspoon beetroot powder

Berry: ½ to ¾ teaspoon alkanet root powder

Coral: 2 drops of natural liquid yellow food color and 3 drops of red

Brown: ½ teaspoon cocoa powder

Alternatively, you can add a bit of your favorite lipstick shade to the lip balm mix. This will result to a sheerer version of your favorite lip color. This is also a great way to save broken lipstick bullets.

Shimmer lip balm

You can add shimmer to clear or tinted lip balm. Use only a pinch of shimmer per batch. Take note that too much shimmer on the lips can look tacky especially on older women. Here are some combinations that look sophisticated.

For clear lip balms: silver or gold mica

For pink and berry tinted lip balm: silver or pink mica

For red and maroon tinted lip balm: copper or gold mica

For coral and caramel tinted lip balm: yellow or gold mica

For brown tinted lip balm: gold mica

<u>Flavored lip balm</u>

Regarding flavors, you can be as simple or as wild as you want. Here are some ideas to get your creative juices flowing.

Honey lemon lip balm

2 tablespoons olive oil

2 teaspoons beeswax pellets

1 teaspoon honey

10 to 15 drops lemon essential oil (use more or less depending on how lemony you want it to be)

Melt the beeswax and olive oil and mix well. Take the mixture off the heat then stir in the honey. When slightly cool, add the lemon essential oil. Pour into your desired containers.

Coconut mango lime lip balm

2 tablespoons coconut oil

2 teaspoons mango butter (another example of an emollient wax, this is made from mango seed)

10 to 15 drops of lime essential oil (use more or less depending on how much lime flavor you want)

Melt the coconut oil and mango butter. Mix well then cool slightly. Add the lime essential oil then pour into your desired containers.

Orange chocolate lip balm

2 tablespoons neutral oil (grape seed, canola, jojoba, or castor)

2 teaspoons cocoa butter

5 drops orange essential oil

5 drops natural chocolate flavor or ½ teaspoon cocoa powder (the latter will give you brown tinted lip balm)

1 drop natural vanilla extract

Melt the oil and cocoa butter. While hot, add the vanilla and chocolate flavor or cocoa powder. Mix well then cool slightly before adding the orange essential oil. Pour into your containers.

Sweet vanilla lip balm

Make a batch of basic moisturizing or protective lip balm. Add ½ teaspoon powdered sugar and ¼ teaspoon vanilla extract.

Spiced grapefruit lip balm

Make a batch of basic moisturizing or protective lip balm. Add ½ teaspoon powdered brown sugar, 5 drops of grapefruit essential oil and 2 drops cinnamon essential oil. (You can make powdered brown sugar by processing brown sugar in a blender or food processor until fine.)

Honey bacon lip balm (if you dare!)

Make a batch of basic protective lip balm. Add ½ teaspoon honey and ¼ teaspoon natural bacon flavor. The honey will make the protective lip balm softer and more emollient.

Anti-aging flavored lip oil

To 2 tablespoons of argan or rosehip oil, add any of the following combinations:

Rose and lemon: 5 drops each of rose and lemon essential oil

Peppermint and grapefruit: 5 drops each of peppermint and grapefruit essential oil

Lavender and honey: 10 drops of lavender and ½ teaspoon honey

Conclusion

Thank you again for reading this book!

I hope this book was able to help you make your own organic lip balms and other lip products.

The next step is to try the suggestions listed here to see what works for you.

Finally, if you enjoyed this book, then I'd like to ask you for a favor, would you be kind enough to leave a review for this book on Amazon? It'd be greatly appreciated!

Thank you and good luck!

Keep reading for a free preview of my book:

*"Ketogenic Diet Cookbook: The Belly Fat Burnin'
Recipe Book for Losing Weight FAST with the
Ketogenic Diet"!*

Chapter 2 - Ketogenic Diet and Weight Loss

The key to successfully applying the ketogenic diet for any budget and personality is by planning ahead. People tend to give up more easily if they do not have a clear set of guidelines to follow. Weight loss, for instance, requires a high amount of willpower.

To begin the keto diet specifically for weight loss, here is a breakdown of the guidelines that you should always keep in mind:

Get rid of all the blatant carbohydrates that you have at home. Donate your breads, cookies, wheat pasta, and other such items to the nearest soup kitchen. Do not even glance at any shop that sells carbohydrates. The following should be banned from your plate (or eaten sparingly, that is to say, a tablespoon per month, maybe) bread, sweets, cereals, potatoes, legumes, beans, and sweet fruit.

Always keep a list of the following food items in your pocket: leafy green vegetables, meats (preferably lean and organic), including beef, fish and other seafood, eggs, chicken, pork, etc., healthy oils and fat (grass-fed butter, coconut, olive, macadamia), cheeses, protein shakes, and nuts. These are the foods that should always be on your plate to provide you with nutrients and energy.

Change your mindset from carb craving to fat and vegetable craving. For example, instead of bread sticks, think of celery sticks; instead of a bagel, try a pork bagel (the recipe is in the next chapter). While many vegetables still have carbohydrates in them, they also contain more fiber and nutrients than any carb-loaded dish out there.

Slowly, but surely, engage in regular workout sessions. Sign up at the gym and have someone guide you from low to high intensity interval workouts. You need to burn off those fat stores as efficiently as you can. Ask about weight training and cardio workouts to boost your metabolism.

Brace yourself for several days (or even weeks) of headaches, nausea, and other symptoms that have to do with the changes that your body is experiencing because of the diet. To prepare for this, make sure to replenish your electrolyte stores. Specifically, these are potassium, sodium and magnesium; these are some of the minerals that your body needs to function properly.

Make sure to read studies and reports about the keto diet so that you can adjust accordingly. Find a reliable online community on the keto diet to share information and meal plans with.

One final tip that you should never forget is to drink plenty of water every day. In a keto diet, you are going to be releasing stored water in your body. You want to catch up with that to avoid dehydration, so make sure to drink lots of water along with electrolytes.

If it is not advisable to do a complete ketogenic diet, you can ask your doctor about the cyclical ketogenic diet instead. In this diet, you are to increase the amount of carbohydrates that you consume in specific meals.

In general, this particular diet entails you to follow the ketogenic diet rigidly for 5 consecutive days, then eat carbohydrate meals in the usual way for 2 days before you go on another 5 days of keto diet. However, this does not mean you should go back to cookies, cakes, and other sugary simple carbohydrates during those 2 days. You should still choose complex carbohydrates such as beans, grains, and vegetables. Keep in mind that the ketogenic diet will not work without exercise, because you still need a means to burn off your fat stores.

Chapter 3 - Breakfast Recipes

Cauliflower Waffles

Makes: 2 waffles

Ingredients:

- 2 eggs
- 1/4 cup mozzarella cheese
- 1/4 cup cheddar cheese
- 3/4 cup coarsely ground cauliflower
- 1 1/2 Tbsp. chopped fresh chives
- 1/4 tsp garlic powder
- 1/4 tsp onion powder
- Red pepper flakes
- Sea salt
- Freshly ground black pepper

Instructions:

1. Place the cauliflower and cheeses in a food processor. Pulse until thoroughly mixed.

2. Add the eggs, chives, garlic and onion powders, and a dash each of red pepper flakes, salt, and black pepper. Process until combined.

3. Pour the mixture into a waffle maker and cook based on manufacturer's instructions.

4. Place waffles on a plate and top with yogurt, cream cheese, and/or crumbled bacon. Serve at once.

If you're interested in checking out the rest of "Ketogenic Diet", then head on over to your closest computer and visit the following link: http://www.books4everyone.com/ketogenic